REIKI 1 MANUAL

EVERYTHING YOU NEED TO KNOW WHEN USING REIKI 1 HEALING

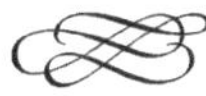

PATRICK HAMOUY

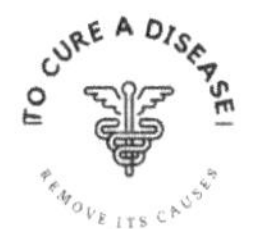

CONTENTS

---

1. https://tomorrowhealthcare.org/contact-query

DISCLAIMER

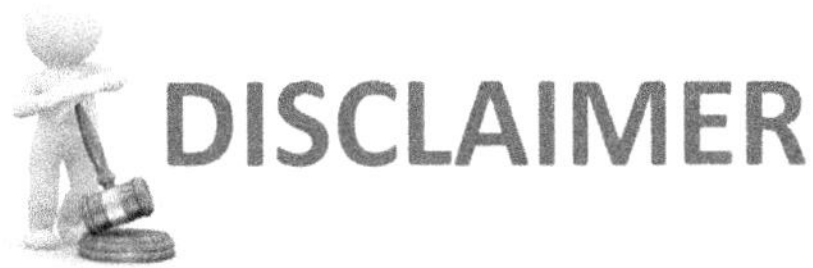

The content of this book is for information only.

The author of this book is not a physician, and the ideas, procedures, and suggestions are not intended to replace trained professionals' medical and legal advice.

All matters regarding your health require medical supervision. Consult your medical practitioner about any condition requiring diagnosis or medical attention.

The author and publishers cannot be held responsible for any errors and omissions found in the text or any actions that a reader may take due to any reliance on the information contained in the text, which is taken entirely at the reader's own risk.

THE ORIGIN OF REIKI

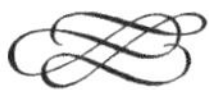

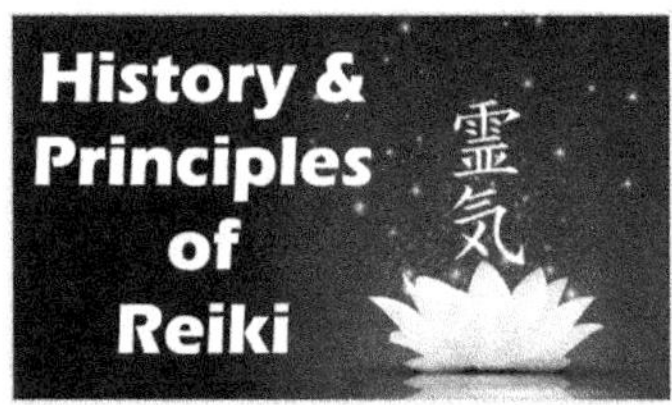

The *origin of Reiki* (pronounced ray-key) is a form of healing that comes to us from Tibet. "The *Healing Buddha"* book is 2,500 years old. It describes a form of healing similar to Reiki. Reiki is passed on from the master to the student. Unless we pass it on, we will lose it. Unfortunately, Dr Mikao Usui, a Japanese Buddhist monk, did not rediscover Reiki until the late 1800s. Reiki is a straightforward technique that anybody may learn.

REI - SPIRITUAL WISDOM

Reiki comes from two Japanese words best translated as "Sharp or Clever spirit."

REI means "The higher intelligence that guides the creation and functioning of the universe".

The direct translation of Rei from a Japanese dictionary is "Ghost".

"Rei" is sometimes translated into "Universal". The meaning of Universal in this context signifies Supernatural Knowledge or Spiritual Consciousness. This wisdom comes from God or the Higher Self. Rei is intelligent; it understands everything. It knows the cause of problems and knows how to deal with them.

KI - THE LIFE FORCE

The direct translation of KI from a Japanese dictionary is Vapour or Mist.

Ki is the Japanese word for Chi in Chinese, Prana in Sanskrit and Mana in Hawaiian. It has also been called Odic force, Orgone, Bioplasma, etc...

Ki is the life energy, often called the Universal Life Force. It is a force that animates all things. All creatures, objects or living things have this life force. The life force flows inside and outside all living things.

It allows us to get up in the morning, work, play, and function as human beings. We feel run down when this life force becomes low, and illness may set in. When this life force flows freely, we are less likely to get sick.

The Ki animates everything we do; it is responsible for our emotions, dreams and daily performance.

Practitioners of Martial arts understand this life force. It has been recognised for at least 4,000 years, as mentioned in the

"*Yellow Emperor's Classic of Internal Medicine*", which lists thirty-two different kinds of Chi.

Spiritually Guided Life Force Energy

Reiki is guided by the God-consciousness called Rei. The practitioner can do very little to influence this energy.

THE FIRST STORY OF REIKI

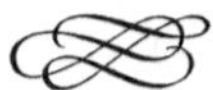

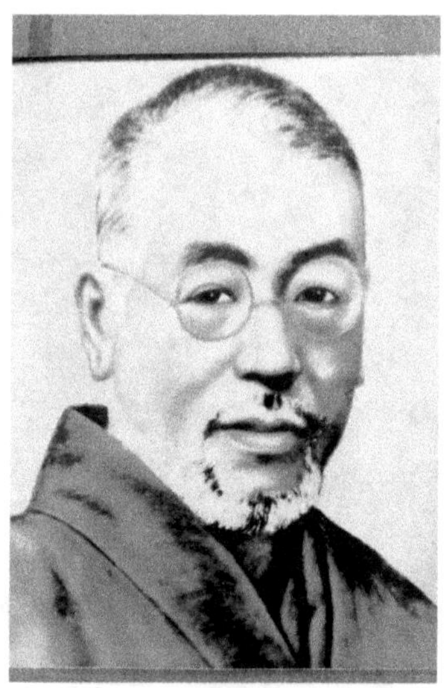

Dr Mikao Usui

There are two different stories about Reiki.

First Story - *Dr Mikao Usui "The Christian Priest"*

Dr Mikao Usui was born in Japan on August 15, 1865, in the village of Yago. He *died on 9 March 1926 of a stroke.* He was married to Sadako Suzuki and had two children.

THE *DOSHISHA UNIVERSITY LETTER*

First, you could get some information on the history of Doshisha University from enclosed photocopies made from Doshisha University Catalogue and The Doshisha.

Second, I, aided by chief archivist, checked the mentioned person, Dr Mikao Usui with the related documents in vain; List of graduate students on Doshisha Alumni Bulletin. Literature relating to J.H. Neesima and List of Faculty and clerical members in those days. I just found out he was never the president of the Doshisha. And the name never appeared, and neither left any trace on them.

So I am afraid I cannot provide any information.

Sincerely,

Itsuro Nishida
Head, Public Services
Center for Academic Information
(formerly Library)
Doshisha University
Kyoto 602 Japan

The original letter from Doshisha University below was very blurry, so I retyped it for you:

First. You could get some information on the history of Doshisha University from enclosed photocopies made from Doshisha University Catalogue and The Doshisha.

Second, I, aided by chief archivist, checked the mentioned person, Dr Mikao Usui with the related documents in vain; List of graduate students on Doshisha Alumni Bulletin. Literature relating to J.H. Neesima, and List of faculty and clerical members in those days. I just found out he was never the president of Doshisha. And the name never appeared, and neither left any traces on them.

So I am afraid I cannot provide you any information.

Sincerely,

Itsuro Nishida
Head, Public Services
Center for Academic Information
(formerly Library)
Doshisha University
Kyoto 602, Japan

Extract from a letter from the University of Doshisha

The blurry letter from Doshisha University

Dr Mikao Usui was the *Principal of Doshisha University*, a Christian school near Kyoto in Japan. It says that one day, his students asked him about healing and asked him to perform some healing tasks. As he could not, he promptly resigned from the school and started his quest for healing.

He is supposed to have travelled to Chicago, where he studied for seven years and received a degree in Technology.

However, a letter from Doshisha University in Japan, where Dr Mikao Usui is supposed to have taught, and a letter from the Divinity School (*Chicago University*) show that Dr Mikao Usui never appeared on their register (the University of Chicago did not even exist in those days).

THE *UNIVERSITY OF CHICAGO LETTER*

THE UNIVERSITY OF CHICAGO
The Office of the University Registrar
CHICAGO, ILLINOIS 60637

November 9, 1990

**Extract from a letter
from the University
of Chicago**

In response to your recent correspondence our records do not indicate that Mikao Usui ever attended the University of Chicago.

I have enclosed our Announcement of the Divinity school.

Maxine H. Sullivan
University Registrar
MHS/mn

THE UNIVERSITY OF CHICAGO ● THE UNIVERSITY OF CHICAGO ● THE UNIVERSITY

The above original letter from Chicago University was very blurry, so I retyped it for you:

It is thought that Mrs *Hawayo Takata* (see her story in the following few pages) believed that if she introduced Dr Usui as a Buddhist monk during the 1940s, nobody would be interested in Reiki. This was too close to Pearl Harbour, and American citizens did not think much of anything or anyone coming from Japan.

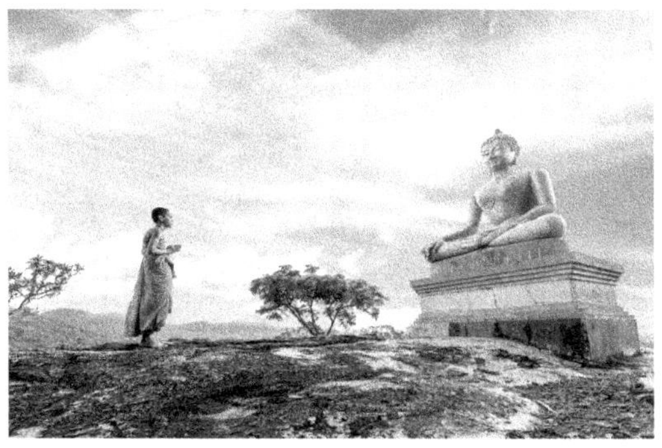

Buddha statue

Dr Usui was interested in Buddha's life and healing. He wondered why Buddha and his disciples could heal physical illnesses and why they lost their power.

As an adult, Dr Usui made it his goal to rediscover how to heal the physical body. He started by visiting Buddhist temples and asking monks if they knew how to heal the physical body. Invariably, the answer was that they did not.

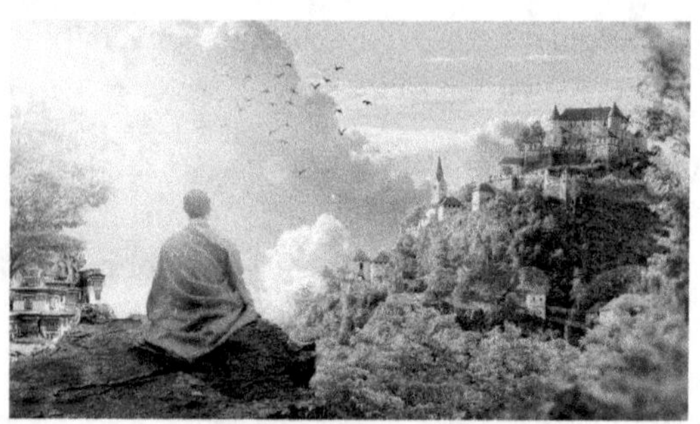

Buddhism Monk Temple

They concentrated on healing the mind, as they believed this was more important, as most diseases came from the mind first.

One of the abbots of a Zen monastery he approached told him that "they no longer knew how to heal the body. They used to, but the skill had been lost through disuse." The abbot was also interested in healing and invited Dr Usui to study with them and look at their secret books in their original language.

To do this, Dr Usui learnt Chinese and eventually Sanskrit. He found part of his answer in the Indian sutras, written in Sanskrit. A formula that allowed him to contact a higher power in meditation.

Armed with this formula, Dr Usui decided to go to the holy *mountain of Koriyama* to *fast and meditate for 21 days.*

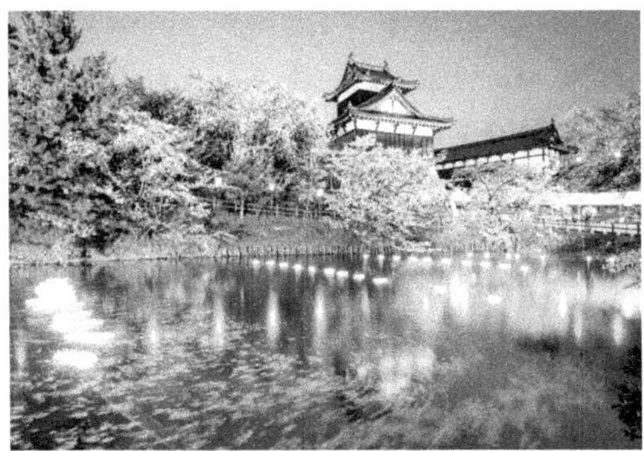

Castle on Koriyama Mountain

He sat on top of the mountain with 21 stones in front of him. Every day as dawn broke, he threw a stone away. He then spent the rest of the day in meditation. On the twenty-first day, he threw his last stone away and shortly after saw a very *bright light on the horizon* coming straight at him.

He realised that this light was a message. He was about to receive what he had been seeking. The light was powerful, and he realised that the light would have to strike him to receive the instructions he needed. This light was mighty, and it might even kill him. Dr Usui was given a choice whether or not he wanted to go through with the experience. He decided to receive the light and see what would happen.

The *light struck him on the third eye* and knocked him unconscious. He then had an out-of-body experience when he saw bubbles of light with symbols. He memorised the signs, and as he did so, he received an attunement so that he was able to use the symbols. This was the way Dr Usui was initiated into Reiki.

When Dr Usui regained consciousness, he was full of energy, although he had not eaten for 21 days. He set out to go back to the monastery, and as he came down the mountain, he tripped, and his toe started to bleed. Instinctively, he rubbed it; the bleeding stopped, and the pain disappeared. He knew then that he had acquired some healing power.

He had a full meal (having fasted for 21 days). He had no adverse effects from this meal (not something I recommend you do even after taking a Reiki course).

Whilst having his meal, he was served by the innkeeper's daughter, who had a terrible *toothache*. Dr Usui felt he could help her and held his hand near her jaw where it hurt. Within a few minutes, the pain had gone.

He discovered that the abbot was in bed, disabled with arthritis at the monastery. He proceeded to relate his experience and, at the same time, successfully treated his friend's problem.

Please note that the above story of the meditation on Mount Koriyama and the subsequent healing only appears in Takata's story. The way Reiki is taught in Japan does not mention these events.

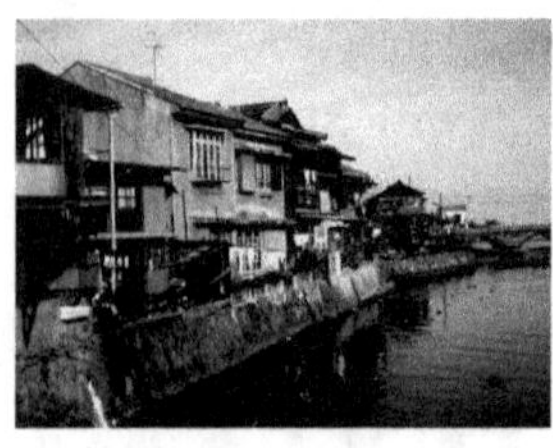

Tokyo's slums

Dr Usui then spent seven years caring for sick people in the slums of Tokyo. Unfortunately, some of these beggars, although cured of physical illnesses, went back to begging, as the life of a working man is much more tiring than begging. Also, without qualifications, it is hard to find work.

Dr Usui realised that he had made a mistake and that the person receiving healing must first ask for it and that there must be an energy exchange. It can be money, work, goods or whatever. Without the person asking for healing or exchanging, he believed the recovery would not work.

Following this realisation, Dr. Usui travelled throughout Japan, seeking healing for individuals in need. He practised and taught Reiki throughout Japan for the remainder of his life. Before his death on 9 March 1926, Usui gave the Master attunement to sixteen teachers, one of whom was Dr Chujiro Hayashi.

Dr *Chujiro Hayashi* is not supposed to have been Dr Mikao Usui's selected Grand Master (Eguchi, who studied with Dr Mikao Usui in 1923, was his chosen successor).

The *Emperor of Japan decorated Dr Usui.* He is buried in a Zen temple in Tokyo.

THE SECOND STORY OF REIKI

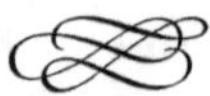

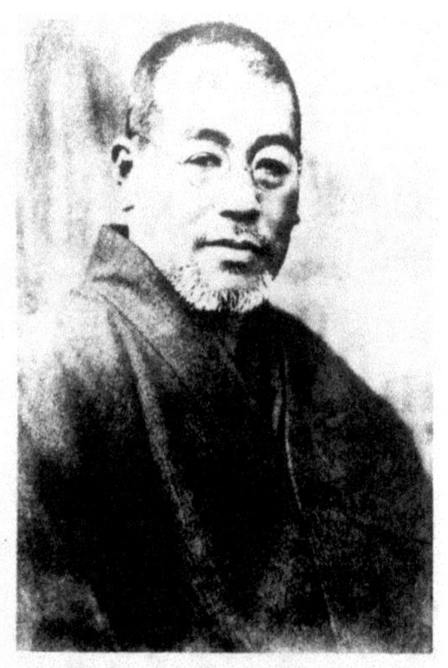

Dr Mikaomi Usui

DR MIKAO USUI "THE BUSINESS MAN"

Reiki originally comes from Buddhist Qigong.

Dr Mikaomi Usui of Kyoto in Japan rediscovered it towards the end of the 19th Century.

DR *MIKAOMI USUI* TRUE STORY

This story comes from Mr *Tsytomu Oishi*, a Japanese gentleman initiated by Mr *Ogawa* in the 1950s. Mr Ogawa was one of Dr Usui's leading students.

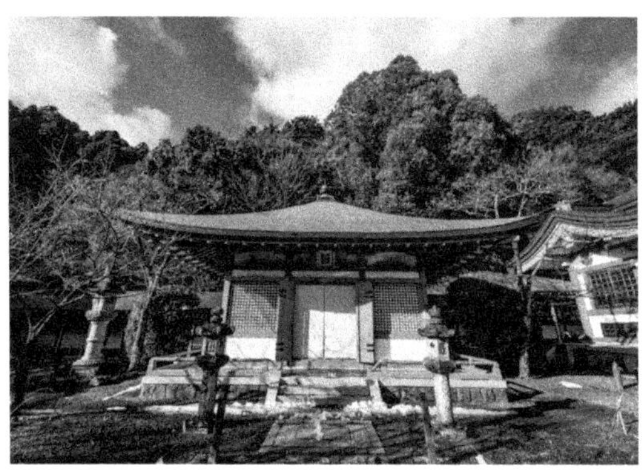

Karuma temple

Dr Usui was born on 15 August 1865, the first year of the Keio Gunnen period. His first name was *Mikaomi,* and his given name was *Gyoho* (it was common practice for a master to provide a new name for their student to create a break between the past and the present).

- *Usui was born in Yago,* a village in southern Japan (in the district of *Yamagata*).
- Usui's *father's name was "Usaemon".*
- *Usui's mother was called "Kawaii".*
- Dr *Usui was married to Suzuki.*
- *Usui and Suzuki had two children together.*

Usui was a hard-working student. As an adult, he travelled west and to China to study.

Usui created a company that went bankrupt. It left him with substantial debts and the desire to get involved in something unrelated to financial gains.

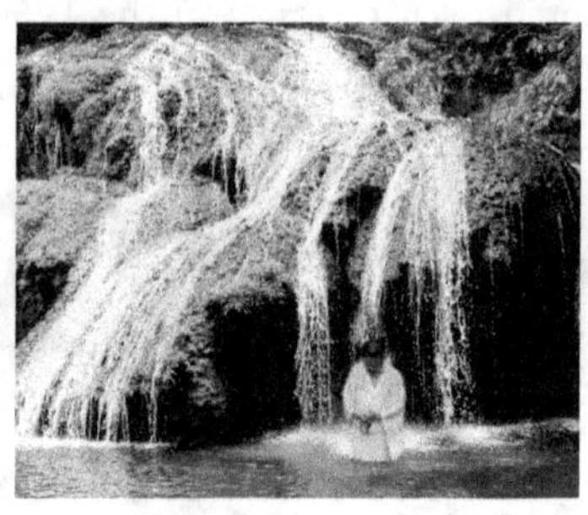

Mount Kurama waterfall

Mount Kurama waterfall is where Usui meditated. One day, he had a *vision* (*satori*) of healing. It probably happened around the years 1918 to 1920. Sometime after this event, he created the "*Usui Reiki Ryoho Gakkai*" (Dr Usui's healing methods).

He first used Reiki on himself and eventually on his family. It worked exceptionally well for all conditions, so he decided to use it on other people.

He opened a *clinic in Harajuku Aoyama, Tokyo, in 1921.* He healed many people and started teaching what he had learnt.

Mr *Kozo,* one of Usui's students, knew instinctively how many sessions were needed to heal a sick person. His Reiki was mighty. Dr Usui acknowledged his accomplishments and elevated him to the highest Reiki ranks.

Usui and Ogawa used to give *crystals charged with Reiki* to their students. Patients were instructed to place these on the body parts that needed healing.

Each new Reiki student was given a complete Reiki manual. This manual describes the standard hand positions and provides information on treating different diseases. Students were not requested to memorise what was taught during the courses.

The "*Usui Reiki Ryoho Gakkai*' was created by Dr Usui, who became its first president. This society's headquarters are still in Tokyo. The *presidents were*:

1. M. Usui (1865–1926)
2. Ushida Juzaburō
3. Taketomi Kan'ichi
4. Watanabe Yoshiharu
5. Wanami Hōichi
6. Koyama Kimiko
7. Kondō Masaki
8. Takahashi Ichita, president, elected in 2010

This society is still active in Japan. The Reiki taught in Japan is similar to the one introduced in Europe. In 1923, *Kanto's earthquake* killed thousands and injured many.

Dr Usui worked relentlessly to help the victims. In February 1924, he built a new *clinic in Nakano near Tokyo*. His fame spread across Japan, and he was in high demand.

Dr *Usui died, aged 61, from a stroke on 9 March 1926* whilst visiting Fukuyama.

DR HAYASHI

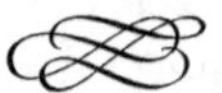

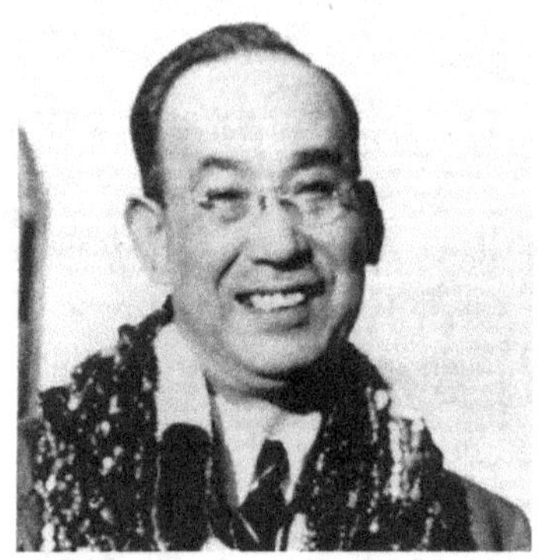

Dr Hayashi

Dr *Hayashi (1880 - 1940), a retired naval officer,* was interested in Dr Usui's work. Dr Usui initiated Dr Hayashi as a Reiki Master.

Dr *Hayashi was initiated as a Master in 1925, aged 47.*

Dr *Hayashi divided Reiki into three degrees* and established new hand positions. Until then, Reiki was given in a series of attunements and could be delivered quickly.

Dr Usui may have been given Reiki in one attunement.

Dr Hayashi opened a Reiki clinic in Tokyo, near the Imperial Palace, and kept detailed records of the treatments given.

His clinic consisted of a reception room and a large room with eight couches and 16 practitioners working (2 per patient). The practitioners worked there from 7 to 12.00 and did house calls until 7 p.m.

Dr Hayashi designed the hand position system taught during the first degree and their initiation procedures.

Hayashi forced his death by mentally rupturing the arteries to his heart on May 10, 1941. Dr Hayashi initiated 13 masters (including his wife) during his lifetime.

One of Hayashi's students was a lady called *Hawayo Takata.*

HAWAYO TAKATA

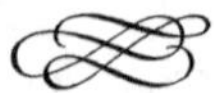

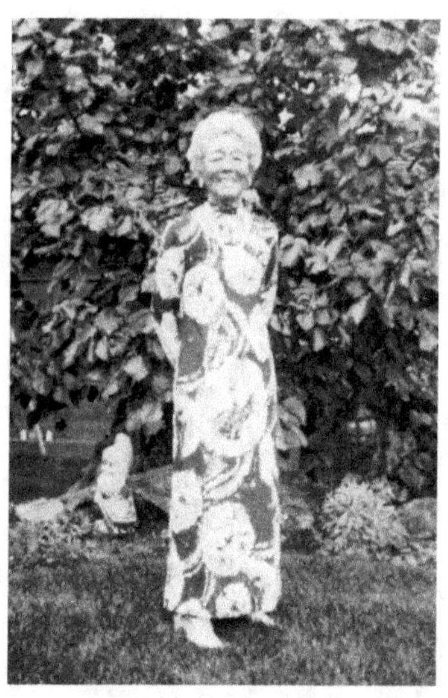

Hawayo Takata was born on 24 December 1900 in Kauai, one of the Hawaiian islands. She was of Japanese origin, and her father worked in a local sugar plantation. She married Saichi Takata, the bookkeeper of the sugar plantation, where she eventually worked herself.

Takata's husband died in October 1930, aged 34, leaving his wife and two children.

Takata took over the family's keeping and eventually suffered from a nervous breakdown, abdominal pains and lung problems.

When her sister died, she went to Japan, where her parents lived, to inform them of the loss of their daughter. She went to the hospital, was diagnosed with a terminal illness, and was rushed for surgery.

> **Author's note**: Specific details about her terminal illness are not documented or publicly confirmed in the historical or Reiki literature.

Whilst waiting for the surgeon, she is supposed to have heard a voice that said:

"The *operation is not necessary*"

She wondered if she was dreaming, but she realised that she was fully awake.

To the staff's surprise, she got off the operating table in the operating theatre, searched for the surgeon, and asked him if he believed there might be an alternative way to resolve her issues instead of undergoing surgery. The doctor told her about Hayashi's clinic.

Takata underwent a course of treatments at Hayashi's clinic. The Reiki practitioners described her symptoms accurately by laying their hands on her. It impressed Takata and gave her the confidence to proceed with the treatment.

She was curious about the heat she received whilst the two practitioners treated her, and thought they might use some *heating apparatus*. She looked under the couch and found nothing. Then she grabbed one of the practitioners' sleeves, thinking some heating equipment was hidden. The startled practitioner laughed at her when she explained what she sought. He told her about Reiki and how it worked.

As she progressed with her daily treatment, her condition got progressively better. She decided that she also would like to learn Reiki.

In a country where a man was king and Japanese pride was high, she was told that Reiki should stay in Japan and that she could not be initiated. Takata was a stubborn person who did not take no for an answer. She asked her surgeon for a letter confirming that she was sick and needed Reiki daily.

Eventually, Dr Hayashi initiated Takata as follows:

> *Takata was initiated into Reiki 1 in 1936.*

> *Takata was formed in the Second Degree in 1937.*

She returned to Hawaii in the summer of 1937 and invited Dr Hayashi's daughter over. She knew that Dr Hayashi would never permit his daughter to travel alone and that there was a good chance he would come with her and possibly initiate her into a Grand Master.

Takata was initiated as a Master on February 21, 1938. Hayashi registered her Master's Certificate in Honolulu, which gave her the right to practice and teach in the United States (only). Her Reiki Master's certificate shows her as a Master (not a Grand Master).

Between 1970 and her death on 11 December 1980, Mrs Takata initiated the following *Reiki Masters:*

1. George Araki
2. Barbara McCullough
3. Beth Gray
4. Ursula Baylow
5. Paul Mitchell
6. Iris Ishikura
7. Fran Brown
8. Barbara Weber Ray
9. Ethel Lombardi
10. Wanja Twan
11. Virginia Samdahl
12. Phyllis Lei Furumoto
13. Dorothy Baba
14. Mary McFadyen
15. John Gray
16. Rick Bockner
17. Bethel Phaigh
18. Harry Kuboi
19. Patricia Ewing
20. Shinobu Saito
21. Takata's Sister
22. Barbara Brown
23. Phyllis Furumoto

PHYLLIS FURUMOTO

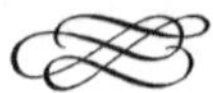

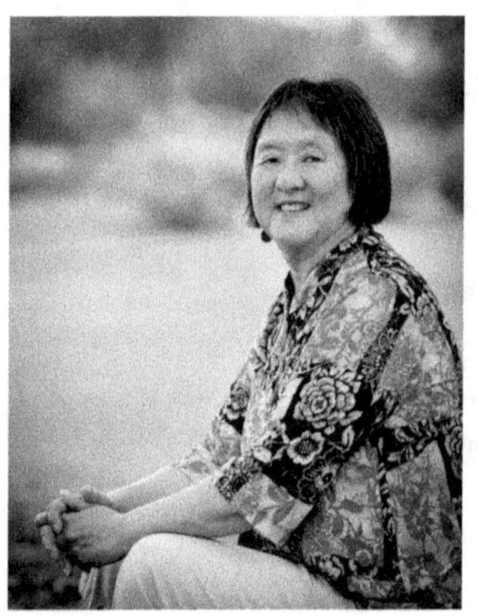

Phyllis Furumoto

Phyllis Furumoto is Takata's granddaughter. Before her death, Takata asked Phyllis if she wanted to become the new Grand Master. Phyllis, at the time, turned the offer down as she was busy playing some sport. 😬

Takata asked Barbara Ray to become the new Grand Master, and Barbara accepted.

Phyllis changed her mind, and Takata initiated her as the new Grand Master without telling Barbara Ray. As you can imagine, this caused some friction...

A STORY INVOLVING PHYLLIS FURUMOTO

Many years ago, I joined a master's group to listen to Phyllis for five days. The trip involved a substantial attendance fee, a fairly long journey, and hotel accommodation.

On the second day, Phyllis announced that she was feeling unwell and would take a few days off to recover. Clever masters present started speculating about what caused her to be unwell. They shared good and crazy ideas.

Eventually, Phyllis came back on day five. 😠

Philis Furumoto was born on August 22, 1948, in Dallas, Texas. She died on March 31, 2019.

BARBARA RAY

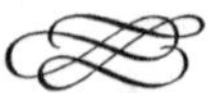

BARBARA RAY AND THE RADIANCE TECHNIQUE

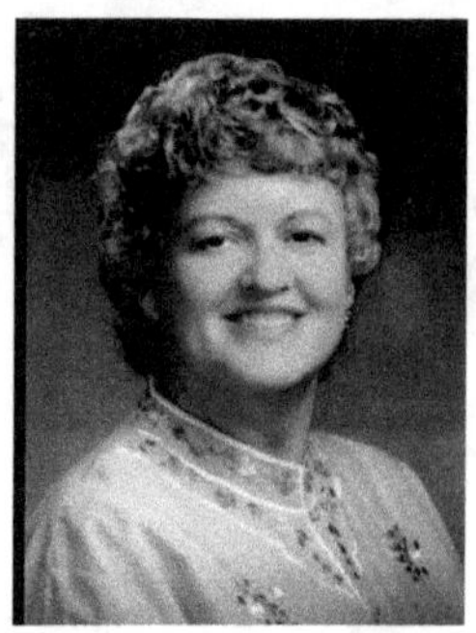

Barbara Ray formed her own Reiki system of healing, initially called:

A.I.R.A - American International Reiki Association

This was later renamed "The *Radiance Technique*". Barbara initially added three new levels to the Reiki natural healing system, followed by a further seventh. Each time, students had to pay to get to the next level. The Radiance technique has now almost disappeared.

VIRGINIA SAMDAHL

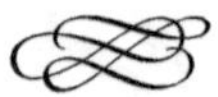

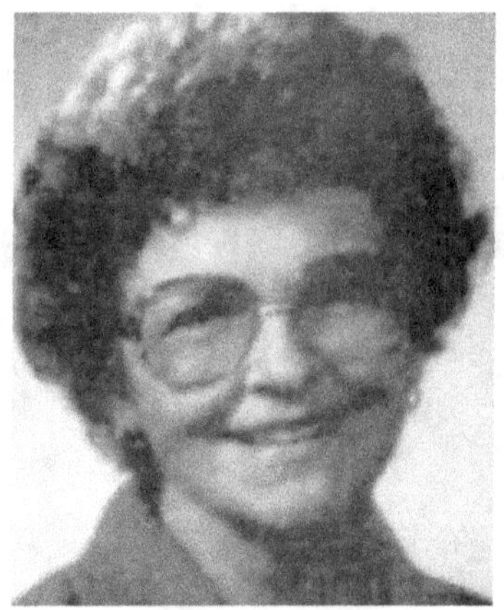

Sorry, I could not find a bigger picture of Virginia
Samdahl

VIRGINIA SAMDAHL

Virginia Samdahl was initiated by Takata in 1974.

She was the first Occidental Reiki master.

THE REIKI ALLIANCE

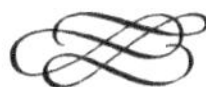

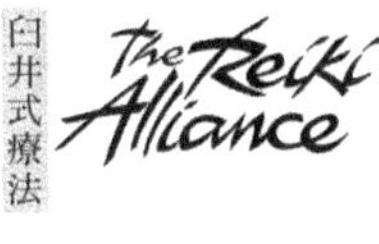 A group of Reiki Masters formed the *Reiki Alliance* in May 1983. It has a set of guidelines on how masters should teach Reiki. The Alliance itself did not teach Reiki. It recognises independent Reiki Masters.

The word Reiki in Japan is used to describe any system of healing. Dr Usui's healing method is:

"The *Usui System of Natural Healing*" or "*Usui Shiki Ryoho*".

Since <u>Dr Usui, Dr Hayashi, or Takata supposedly did not leave any written records</u>, we rely on what was passed on from Master to students.

Initially, Reiki was not so structured. Dr. Usui received Reiki in one powerful attunement and initiated his students quickly. The Alliance has established a required waiting period between each level of Reiki training.

After his experience with the beggars in the slums of Tokyo, Dr. Usui added that one needs to give something in exchange for Reiki. It could be money, work, or anything else, depending on the person's financial means. Dr. Hayashi introduced the hand position, and *Takata added the fee structure.*

Many new Masters have made changes to the way they teach Reiki. Some of these changes are beneficial, while others are not.

Barbara Ray, for example, introduced four new levels to Reiki. During their initiations, her students no longer received the names of the secret symbols. She changed the name of Reiki to Radiance Techniques.

THE $10,000.00 FEE

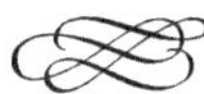

As previously mentioned, Mrs. Takata introduced the $10,000 fee around 1970.

She believed that *Japanese people have different values* from ours. For example, many Japanese people worked for the same company for most of their lives and had values that are rare in the West.

She wondered how to earn the respect of aspiring Western Reiki masters. She decided that Westerners respected money and fixed a fee of $150 for Reiki 1, $500 for Reiki 2, and $10,000 for Reiki 3.

$10,000 in 1970 is equivalent to approximately $81,000 in 2025.

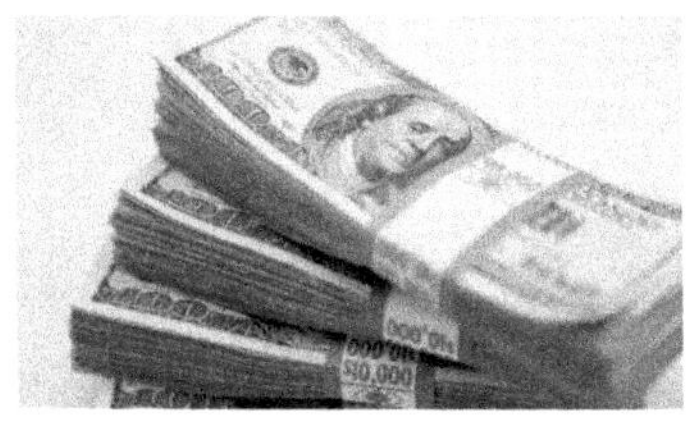

I don't believe any Alliance Reiki Masters still charge these fees. This code of conduct does not bind independent teachers, allowing them to charge significantly lower fees.

This, in turn, will mean more Masters become available. These changes will contribute to more people learning Reiki and a healthier planet, with more people taking their health into their own hands.

DR. MIKAO USUI & THE REIKI IDEALS

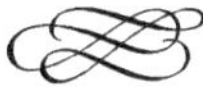

Several years after his mystical experience on Mt. Kori-Yama, Dr. Usui received these Reiki Ideals during a meditation session. These ideals became the foundation of his teachings, guiding practitioners along a path of spiritual growth and self-improvement. They force the person to think about their problems and do something positive to eliminate them.

JUST FOR TODAY, DO NOT WORRY

Just for today, do not worry

Just for today, do not anger

Honour your parents, teachers and elders

Earn your living honestly

Show gratitude for everything

We all know that worrying is futile. It does not solve any problem. Working on a problem will solve it. Worrying about it will magnify it and make it more powerful. The meaning here is that if you encounter a problem, please take action to address it. Please address the issue and resolve it if possible. Avoid worrying about it, as it does not help.

Worrying also indicates a lack of understanding that everything in life has a purpose. When problems arise, we often feel that they are unfair and question why they happen to us. With time, we may discover that what seemed to have been a terrible patch was a positive turning point in our lives. We may have followed a different path that provided more fulfilment and happiness than we previously had. Please consider your past challenges; you may find one that aligns with what I'm referring to.

Nobody is perfect. Your imperfections do not matter and are acceptable as long as they do not cause harm to others. This promotes the idea of self-acceptance and encourages individuals to focus on their intentions rather than striving for unattainable perfection.

"Expect the best in life, and when you receive something you did not expect, know that it is the best for you in your present situation."

JUST FOR TODAY, DO NOT ANGER

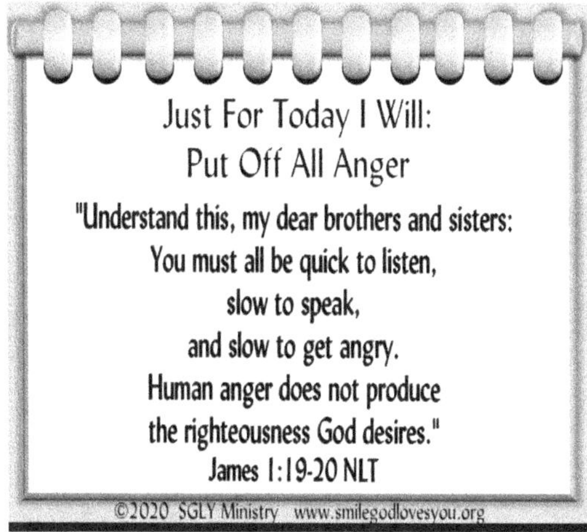

It is not meant to imply that if you are angry, you are evil. The idea is to avoid harbouring anger. It is OK to rage, but then you must let it go. Anger will otherwise affect your liver.

HONOUR YOUR PARENTS, TEACHERS AND ELDERS.

Be grateful for the lessons you learn. You can learn something from virtually everybody.

SHOW GRATITUDE TO EVERYTHING

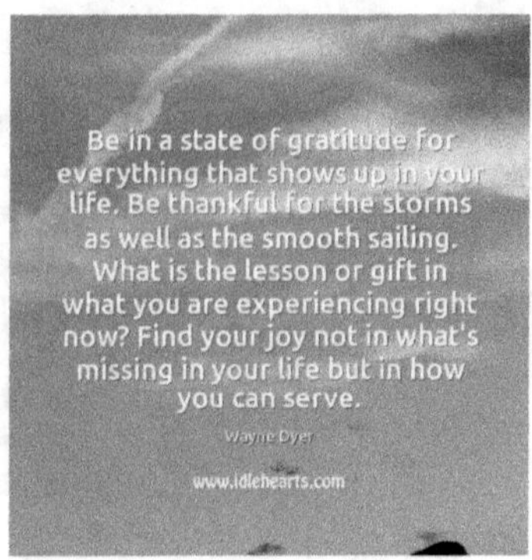

To live in gratitude is to live in abundance.

Being grateful for everything that happens to you means living in happiness.

EARN YOUR LIVING HONESTLY

You must not suppose,
because I am a man of
letters, that I never tried to
earn an honest living

George Bernard Shaw

PICTUREQUOTES.com

Be honest with yourself first. You may cheat others, but you cannot fool yourself.

When we face life honestly, we can see the lessons.

Life of illusion is very complex.

You will project honesty onto others and reap rewards if you are honest with yourself.

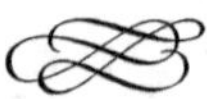

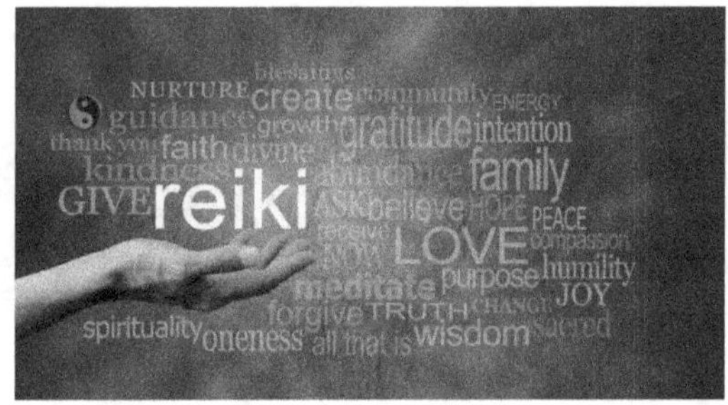

Reiki has spread rapidly. It is now practised in most countries around the world. In 1992, there were an estimated 800 Reiki Masters, with as many as 60,000 people practising Reiki worldwide.

Estimated Number of Reiki Masters Worldwide (as of 2025):

Over 1 million Reiki Masters globally.

Tens of millions have received at least Reiki Level 1 attunement.

IS *REIKI THE ONLY FORM OF HEALING?*

Reiki is not the only form of healing. All healers use KI, but not all use Rei Ki. Reiki healing is different in several aspects:

- Reiki is intelligent. You do not need to guide Reiki to certain parts of your patient's body. Reiki will go where it is required. Reiki is more powerful when hand treatment is given directly over areas where pain or a problem exists.
- You do not need a physical or mental ability to learn Reiki. Anybody can learn Reiki. Children can remember the first degree from when they understand about hurts and healing.
- Giving Reiki does not drain your energy, but rather replenishes it. When giving Reiki, you are not using your energy; you are receiving universal energy, which is channelled through you and passed on to your patient. When you give the treatment, you shall receive energy if you need power. This is a good reason to always be willing to give Reiki.

You can *learn the different levels of Reiki in two weekends* (i.e., one weekend for Reiki 1 and one for Reiki 2). There is no need to learn difficult and complex procedures.

A master passes Reiki to a student. It always works as long as the master is genuine. The guide who initiates ensures that the person has Reiki after the attunement.

Reiki remains with you for life.

If your *Reiki is not used for a long time, you may lose it*.

If the person receiving the Reiki attunement is already a healer, it will at least *double their current healing powers*.

You do not have to enter an altered state when giving Reiki. Simply thinking of Reiki or saying a silent prayer and asking Reiki to flow in you is sufficient to start Reiki.

Once Reiki has begun, you do not specifically need to concentrate on what you are doing, although this seems to increase its effectiveness.

Reiki can never cause harm. Do not worry about giving Reiki. It is always helpful.

THE ATTUNEMENTS

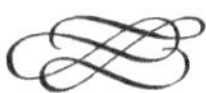

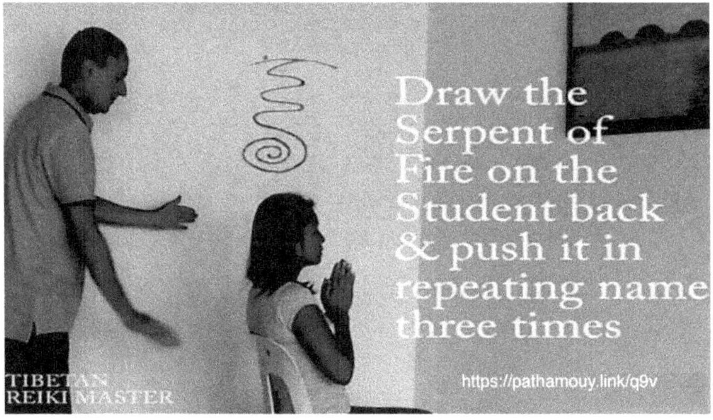

If you are interested in initiating students, please check our Reiki movie for ALL attunements [1].

A *master passes on Reiki to a student* during a series of initiations. The *initiations open the crown, heart, and palm chakras* where the Reiki energy can flow.

---

1. https://tomorrowhealthcare.org/reiki-initiation-tutorial-movie

It is not unusual for students to have memorable experiences during the attunement. Many reports *seeing purple, white, or green colours*; some have visions or are given messages, etc.

Spiritual Reiki guides carry out the Reiki attunements through the master. They are responsible for overseeing the initiation process and are aware of each student's specific requirements. The initiation might enhance your psychic sensitivity or intuition and open your third eye.

21-DAY SELF-TREATMENT

After receiving a Reiki attunement, you should treat yourself with Reiki for 21 days. It is known as the:

21-day cleansing process

This cleansing process operates not only on the body but also on the mind. Therefore, it is not unusual for people's moods to change as the process is happening. Past illnesses may flare up for a short time and then disappear. It is known as a healing crisis.

YIN/YANG NATURE OF REIKI

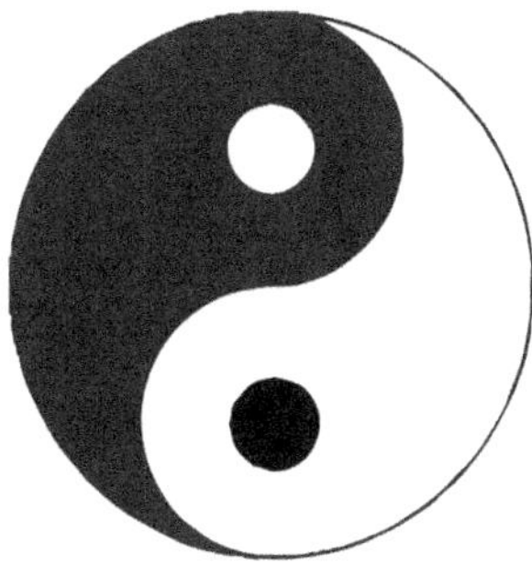

Yin Yang symbol

Like the macrobiotic system of medicine, Reiki works on a male/female energy system. The male (Yang) part comes from the Crown Chakra (called Shiva in the Tantra system), and the female part (Yin) comes from the Base Chakra (called Shakti in the Tantra system). This energy combines in your body to create balance, even if several Reiki healers are working on it simultaneously.

HOW DOES REIKI WORK?

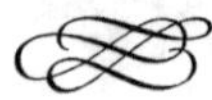

The *effects of a Reiki treatment are as follows:*

1. *Energy balancing*
2. *Awareness increase*
3. *Whole person healing*
4. *Energy amplification*
5. *Reiki works on the causal level of disease*
6. *Stress release*
7. *Emotion release*
8. *Creativity increase*

As previously mentioned, the Reiki practitioner is not responsible for generating Reiki energy. It is provided to them by higher spiritual guides.

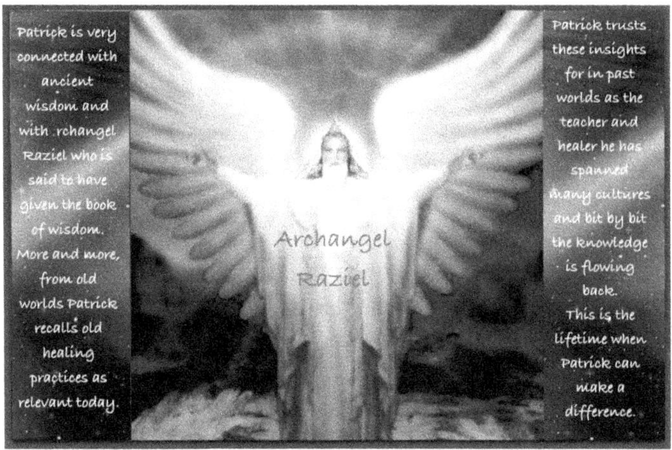

Patrick's guide Archangel Raziel

Reiki replenishes the energy in us that we need to function during the day. This energy allows us to get up, work, play, and do whatever we want during the day. When we deplete this energy, we experience fatigue and become more vulnerable to illnesses.

Negative messages or poor diets eventually deplete our energy, leading to illness.

SOME *STATISTICS*

A US survey found that kids received 434 negative and 23 positive messages daily. Therefore, it is hardly surprising that their energy flow becomes negative.

Reiki is a bit like charging a battery. It boosts our energy when it is low and allows us to regain health.

MY CLAIRVOYANT FRIEND

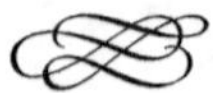

MY CLAIRVOYANT FRIEND

A few years ago, I gave Reiki to a friend with knee pain. This friend has been a *clairvoyant and natural healer from birth*. I explained how Reiki worked, and as she was a clairvoyant, I suggested that she go into a trance and try to communicate with the higher guide performing the healing on her.

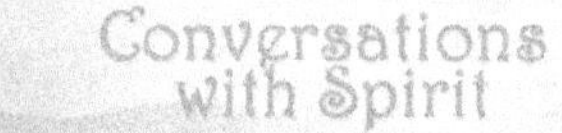

She did, and for a couple of hours, we had a three-way *conversation where I could talk to my guide*, ask questions, and be given the answer by my friend.

It was one of the most exciting experiences I have ever had. During the conversation, my friend told me that the guide was leaving her to perform some work on me, as he (my guide, who showed himself as a male) had realised that I had pain in my descending colon. The guide said that the pain was due to a slight twist in the colon, and he would stretch it.

My abdomen made a gurgling noise, and all pain stopped. I was impressed, as I had not even told my friend about the pain.

Since then, I have used my guide(s) to assist me in my practice and in treating my clients. I was amazed at the accuracy of the diagnosis given.

CONTRA-INDICATIONS - WHAT CAN BE TREATED?

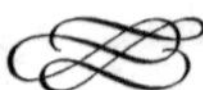

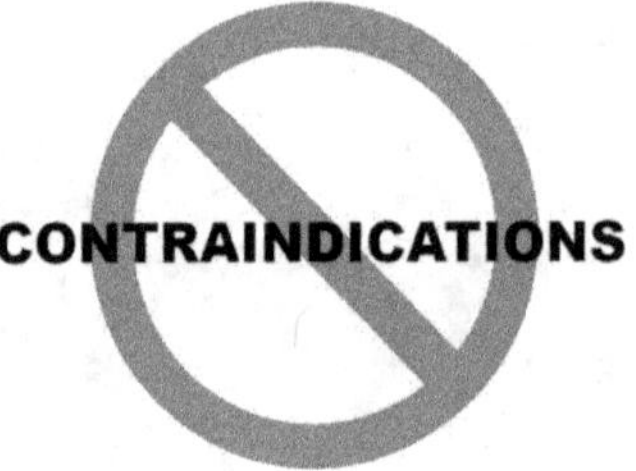

As a practitioner, you should always recommend that your patients *consult a doctor for a medical condition.*

There are a few *contraindications to Reiki:*

- When treating a broken leg, the bone must be set before you treat; otherwise, the healing may start too soon with the bone in the wrong place.
- Suppose you have a problem with the electrical current (i.e., one of our tutors regularly blew up our bulbs when switching the lights on at the school). I advised her not to work with anybody with a

pacemaker or a battery-operated machine on their body.

- You cannot give Reiki to somebody under anaesthetic as this may cancel the drug's effect.
- It is best not to treat psychotic patients, as it may accelerate the onset of the disease. Reiki does not cause this; it only makes it happen quicker.

You can treat any other condition. There are numerous accounts of patients successfully overcoming conditions such as cancer, heart issues, ME, MS, AIDS, and more.

WORKING ON PLANTS AND ANIMALS

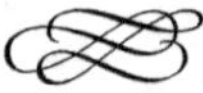

WORKING ON PLANTS

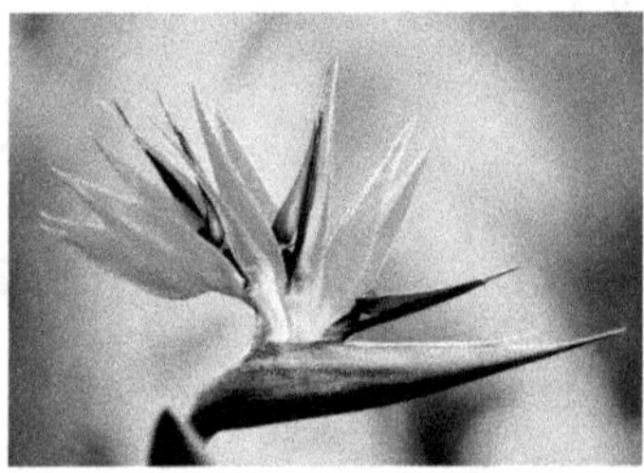

I did not Reiki this plant, but it is beautiful

When using Reiki, a practitioner can work as efficiently on plants as they can on animals. I bought two similar plants as an experiment at the start of my Reiki training. I positioned them next to each other to have equal exposure to the sun and the external environment. I gave each plant the same amount of water regularly. The plant I treated with Reiki soon blossomed into a much prettier plant than the other one.

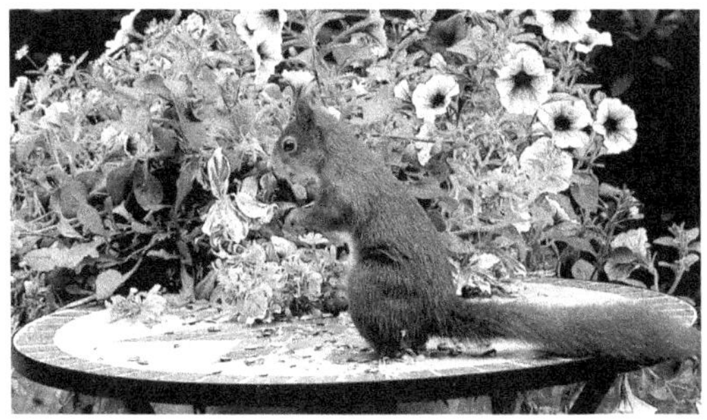

WORKING ON ANIMALS

Animals will also respond to Reiki. I have tried this numerous times on my cat and other animals. Animals are much more sensitive to Reiki energy and seem to feel it more readily than some humans.

One amusing story is that of a dog that hurt his leg and developed a severe limp. His owner gave the dog Reiki, and the leg got better. Since then, each time the dog wants Reiki, he walks with a limp.

Reiki is not a religion. People from different races and religions can practice it.

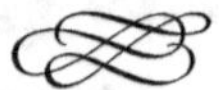

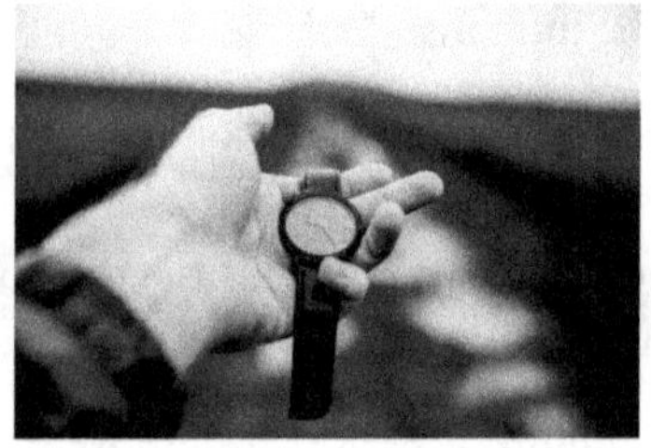

You sometimes can fix a broken watch with Reiki

You may also use *Reiki to work on broken objects*. For example, it has repeatedly repaired watches, radios, calculators, etc.

Reiki also helps recharge batteries in a car or any object with batteries.

HOW TO GIVE A REIKI TREATMENT

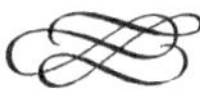

If you offer *Reiki treatments* to customers, friends or family, you should invest in a good **couch.**[1]

To start Reiki, the only thing you need to do is intend to give Reiki. You may, if you wish, *murmur a prayer* and specify which specific problem you want to treat.

You do not need to enter a meditative state to give Reiki. You may talk to the client during the treatment. However, your Reiki will be stronger if you concentrate and try visualising the energy healing your patient.

---

1. https://ebay.us/FvzbyA - Ebay link for couches

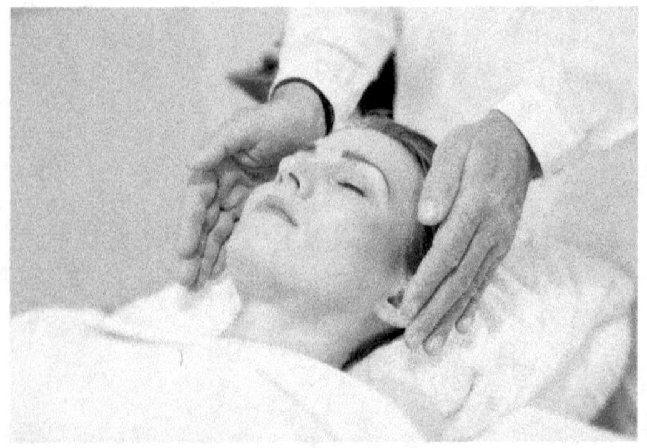

Treat the *customer's aura* for a few minutes at the beginning of the treatment. You should keep your *fingers together* when giving a treatment. It concentrates the energy.

The complete body *treatment should last about 1 hour.*

You may give Reiki for more extended periods. You may spend several *hours working on a patient daily* without fear of overdosing. *Reiki is intelligent;* it knows where to direct the energy in the patient.

Treatments may last a few minutes. It does not need to be a full hour. Whatever you do, Reiki will help.

Different *sensations may be felt in your hands* (tingling, heat, cold, pain, pulsation, etc.). You may also feel joy, love, freedom, etc.

Let your *intuition guide you when giving Reiki.* The standard hand positions are only there to help you. If you feel the patient needs healing on the elbow (not on the regular hand positions), go for it.

Remember that whilst giving Reiki, you are also receiving Reiki.

STEPS TO FOLLOW FOR A COMPLETE REIKI TREATMENT

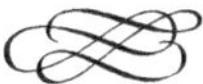

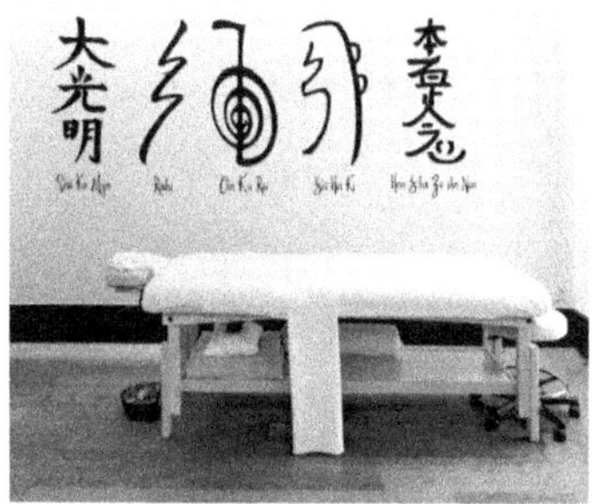

PREPARE FOR A COMPLETE *REIKI TREATMENT*

- Prepare the room before the client comes.
- Make sure the room is warm enough.
- Have a **couch**[1] or somewhere comfortable for the client to lie. It will save your back and make the treatment much more comfortable for both of you.

---

1. https://ebay.us/FvzbyA

- Wash your hands before and after the treatment.
- Scan your patient's body before the treatment and make a note of sensations.
- Begin the treatment using all the hand positions.
- Try to concentrate on the Reiki energy. It will help.

TREATING SERIOUS AILMENTS

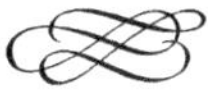

TREATING SERIOUS AILMENTS

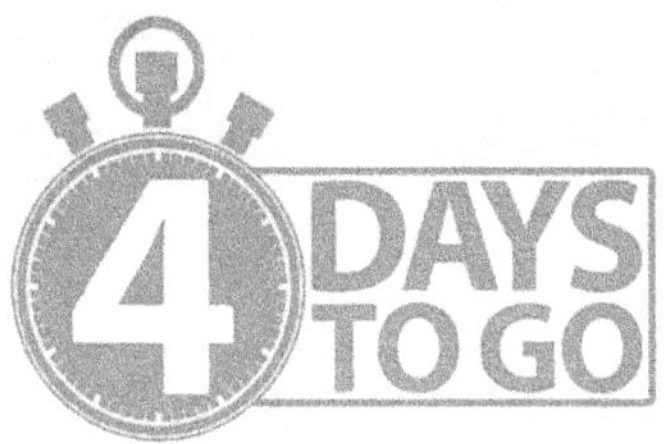

When helping a new patient with Reiki, treat them for four consecutive days for a minimum of 1 hour.

After that, you may treat them once or twice a week, depending on the severity of their condition, and gradually reduce the treatment over several weeks.

HAND POSITIONS TREATING OTHERS

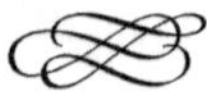

Books and Reiki masters disagree on hand positions to treat others. When treating a person, you must position your hands on all body parts that need to be treated.

For example, if a patient has a problem with their wrist, you must place your hands over their wrist.

You should stay in each position for approximately 3 minutes.

The best way to time yourself is to use our **Reiki with Tibetan Bell music**. The music warns you every three minutes, with the beautiful sound of the Tibetan bell, that it is time to change position.

If you are new to Reiki, you may also like our **Reiki With Instructions Music** (same link as above), **which verbally informs you where to move your hands every three minutes**.

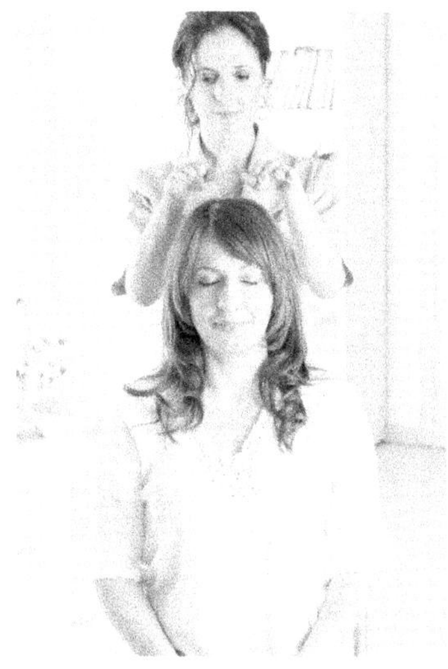

Altogether, I have recorded the following three Reiki MP3s.

1. Meet your Reiki guide
2. Gentle Reiki music with a Tibetan bell sound every three minutes
3. Reiki Music With Hand Position Instructions Every Three Minutes
4. All three Reiki music pieces for a discounted price

You may purchase any or all, these videos here[1].

---

1. https://tomorrowhealthcare.org/reiki-meditations-and-music

SELF-TREATMENT

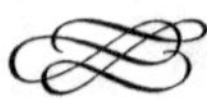

One of the significant advantages of Reiki, as opposed to other healing forms, is that you can treat yourself with Reiki.

As you do not use your energy for treatment, it does not matter how well you feel. You can take care of yourself even when you're feeling down.

HAND POSITIONS FOR TREATING SELF

Use the following hand positions for self-treatment.

Hold each position for approximately three minutes. You can stay in a location as long as you want before moving on.

The best way to time yourself is to use our Reiki with Tibetan Bell music. This warns you every three minutes, with the beautiful sound of the Tibetan bell, that it is time to change position.

If you are new to Reiki, you may also like our Reiki With Instructions Music, which verbally informs you where to move your hands every three minutes.

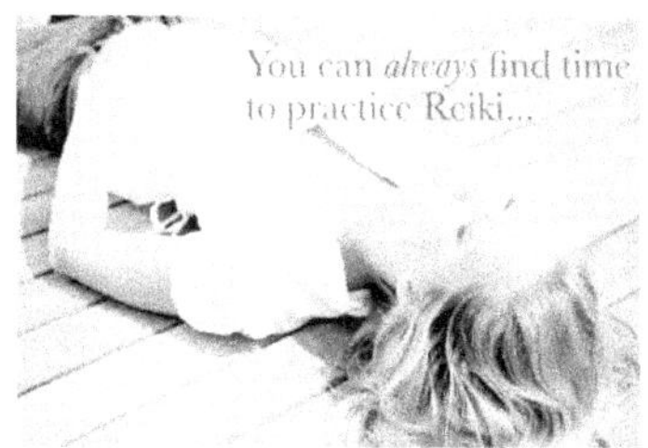

Click here if interested in these recordings[1].

---

1. https://tomorrowhealthcare.org/reiki-meditations-and-music

FINISHING A TREATMENT

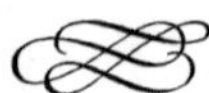

FINISHING A TREATMENT

I always thank my guide for helping me with Reiki at the end of a treatment. I usually ask them to assist this person for another xxx minutes after the end of the treatment. The method works.

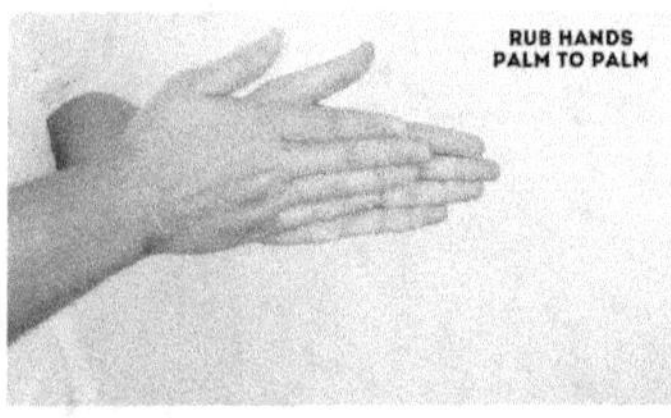

A formal way to end treatment is to rub your hands together and blow on them.

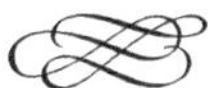

SCANNING

Your Reiki attunement will open the Chakras, increase intuition, and heighten sensitivity to psychic energy. When using the chakras in the palms of your hands, it is possible to sense where the client needs Reiki.

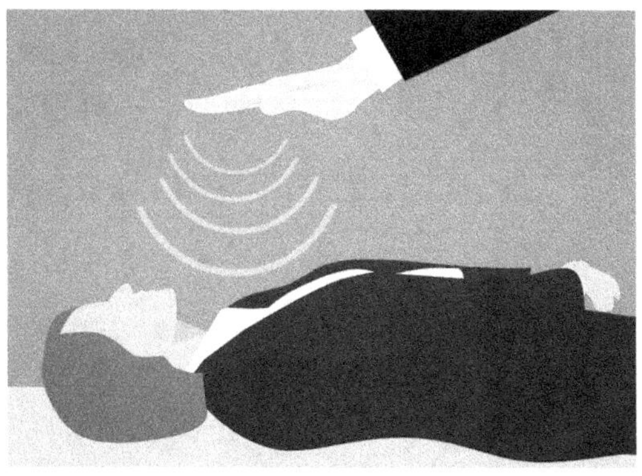

Move your hands slowly over the body

Listen to your hand. Move your hand 1 to 4 inches above the body. *Scan the whole body* moving slowly.

Be aware of different *sensations in your hand*, wrist, arm, and elbow. If one side of your hand hurts, move towards that same side on the patient's body. If the pain suddenly increases and then diminishes, go back to where it was at its peak.

Congratulations, you have located an area of imbalance that needs Reiki. Stay on that area. With some experience, you will learn to recognise when the part of the body you are treating no longer needs more energy.

Carry on scanning until you have scanned the whole body.

Self Scanning

You can also perform self-scanning. The procedure to follow is the same as above. You may find that you are not as sensitive when scanning yourself as when scanning others. This is quite normal.

SCAN FROM A DISTANCE

With experience, you can scan a person far from you, or even a person in a picture or simply in your mind.

WORKING ON THE AURA

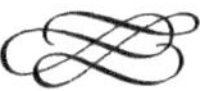

WORKING ON THE AURA

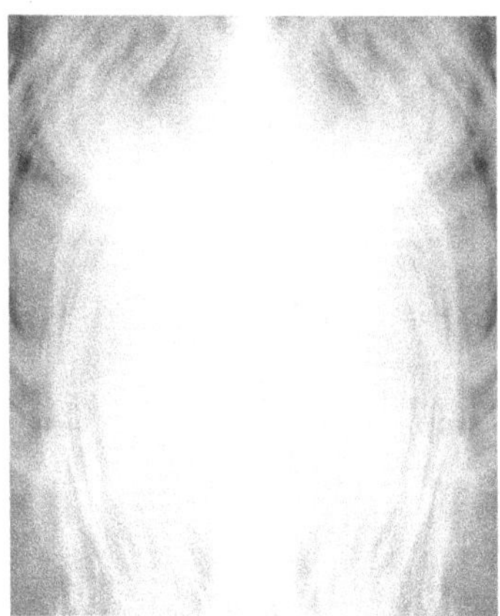

The aura

You may give *Reiki a few inches above the body*. This helps the *etheric field (the aura)* surrounding our body, and is also very useful for emotional problems (and physical problems).

It is helpful when treating people who do not like to be touched or if you do not want to (or cannot because of wounds, burns, etc.) touch your patient.

REIKI 2

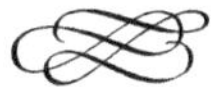

Second-degree Reiki allows you to:

- Send Reiki on a distant basis
- Clear a room of negative energy
- It works on the mental/emotional plane
- It powerfully reinforces a physical healing session
- It works on events past, present, or future
- It heals unwanted habits
- It helps you develop wanted habits, etc.

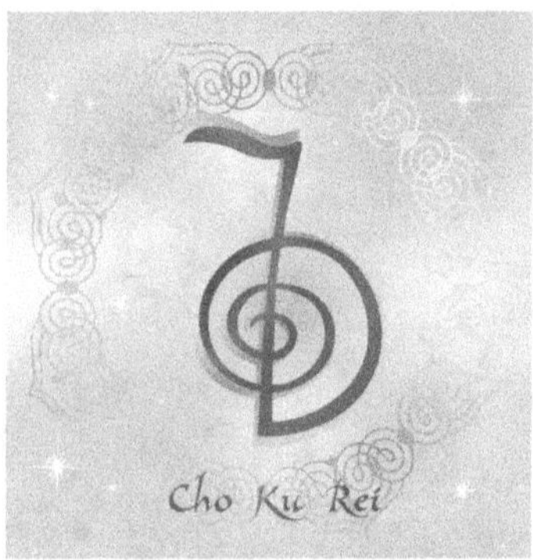

Reiki 2 symbol

You can use three symbols in second-degree Reiki. The first symbol is known as the distant symbol. This symbol lets you send healing to people far away, even in other towns, countries, or planets. Reiki will travel to them and heal them.

The second symbol is called the "*power symbol.*" You can use it to strengthen a physical treatment and enhance its power. You can also use it to clear a room of negative energy or protect yourself against your clients' or others, negative energy.

The *mental/emotional symbol* will allow you to work on emotional traumas. Mind, body, and spirit are closely connected, and sometimes, one cannot heal the body without working on the mind.

The mental/emotional symbol heals the mind. It is a valuable symbol to use in distress, emotional upsets, wanting to eliminate bad habits, or acquiring new (good) behaviours. It also allows you to exorcise possessed souls and helps lost souls on their way to the spiritual world.

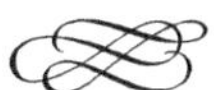

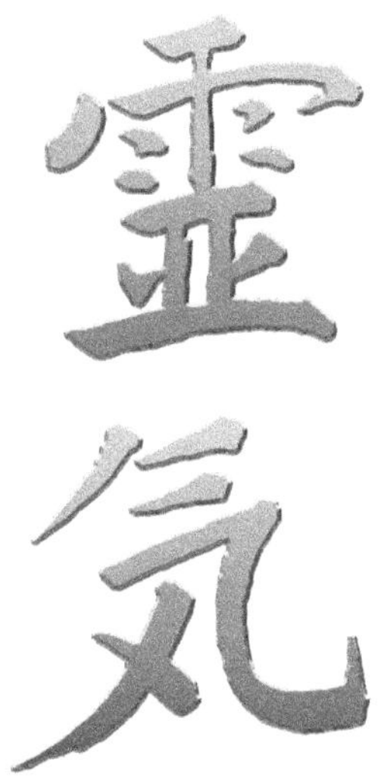

Reiki 3 gives you access to the Master symbol that multiplies the strength of your healing.

This allows you to teach Reiki to other would-be practitioners.

Should you be interested in initiating Reiki students to any level, my video teaches you how to do this[1].

---

1. https://tomorrowhealthcare.org/reiki-initiation-tutorial-movie

ABOUT THE AUTHOR

PATRICK HAMOUY has written several books on natural medicine[1].

Patrick specialises in guiding customers[2] to recover from cancer and other life-threatening diseases using the power of different foods, herbs, detoxification, etc.

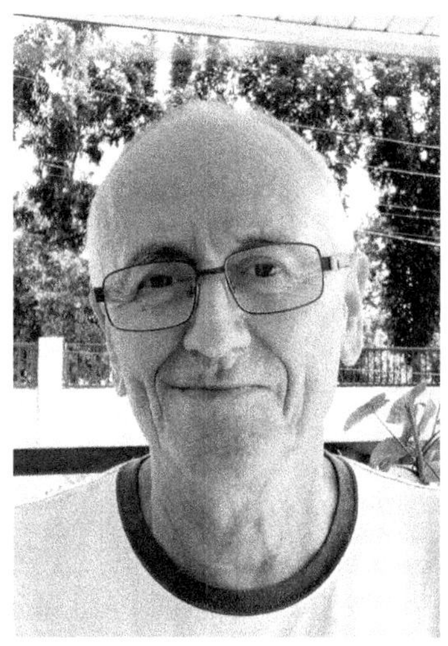

Patrick

In his own words:

In July 1991, my health was feeble after many stressful years

---

1. https://tomorrowhealthcare.org/books
2. https://tomorrowhealthcare.org/full-consultation-with-patrick

running my computer company and a bad diet. I had *cancerous tumours in my liver and colon.*

I was given a *death sentence* by modern medicine.

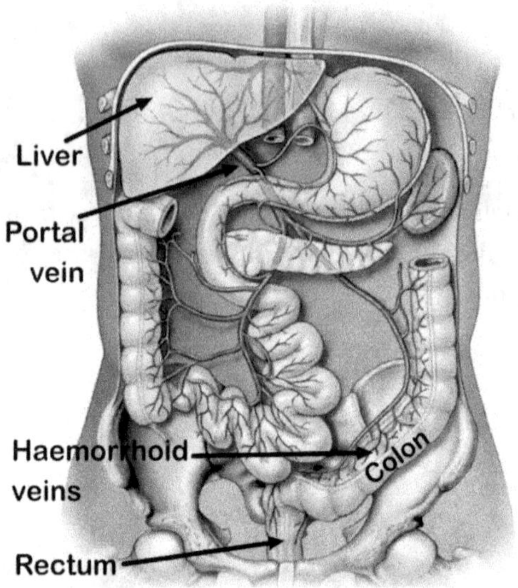

For many years, I had amateurishly tried to take care of my health using natural remedies, and I was fascinated with alternative therapies.

The 1991 recession significantly impacted my computer company, giving me time to study,_as there were no customers in sight. I joined various evening and weekend courses from 1991 to 1993 and qualified in anatomy & physiology, aromatherapy, reflexology, and massage. My health improved slightly, but my cancer still put me on death row.

MY RECOVERY WITH MACROBIOTICS & VEGANISM

In July 1991, I started following a rigorous macrobiotic life-style, which significantly contributed to saving my life.

My macrobiotic and other studies allowed me to learn:

- How different foods in the body can negatively affect our health
- How to use vegetables, fruits, grains, spices, wild foods, and herbs to heal most illnesses (including those classified as "autoimmune")
- The damage caused by negative emotions and excessive stress
- Learn about the diseases caused by the vast number of **poisonous chemicals** in our environment
- Learn about viruses and how to cleanse the body of them. Everybody in the world today has suffered from a virus. Those are escaping modern medicine's detection and weapons.
- How to remove mercury, lead, copper, arsenic, aluminium, nickel, cadmium, other deadly metals, plastics, radiation, chlorine, fluoride, pesticides, herbicides, fungicides, cleaning solvents, etc., from our body as they feed cancers, viruses, and bacteria and cause inflammation.

For many years now, I have moved to a *Vegan diet*[3] that is less restrictive than Macrobiotics.

In mid-1993, I formed my school with a small group of trusted therapists' friends, and we started teaching.

---

3. https://tomorrowhealthcare.org/vegan-diet-benefits

OTHER STUDIES

Helping people get better and recover from all types of so-called incurable diseases has become my way of life.

I joined a multitude of courses on natural medicine over the years. I got fascinated by the power of herbs and supplements to help the body.

I read a couple of hundred books on natural recoveries.

LIFE AFTER MY RECOVERY

Except for a broken bone in my right hand, **I have NOT visited a doctor since July 1991**. As of 2025, I am fit and well.

My Life:

- I was born in France but lived mainly in England—Maidenhead, Gerrards Cross, and Saltdean (a village near Brighton).
- I have two sons: Charles, born in 1986, and Philip, in 1988. They graduated, and both have landed excellent jobs. They live in England.
- I ran my alternative medicine school in the UK between 1993 and 2008.
- I gave lectures on health issues to various individuals and organisations.
- Today, I am fit and healthy. I have not used any drugs or undergone any harmful treatments. I am 74 years old (born 1951).
- In March 2008, I left England to live in the Philippines.

- I give consultations[4] on the internet using FREE communication systems such as <u>Skype</u>[5] or <u>WhatsApp</u>[6].
- In December 2003, I met my wife. We've been together since July 2007. We got married in January 2008. I love her dearly, and she is responsible for my living in the Philippines.

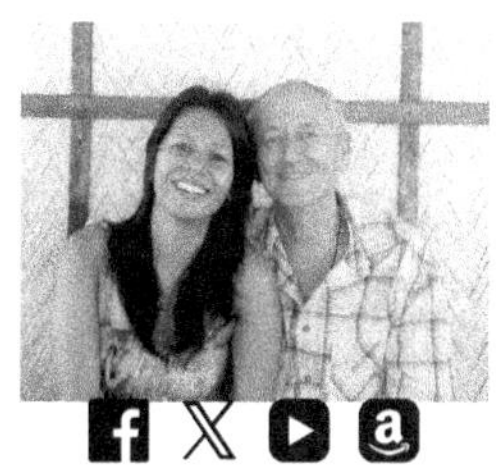

4. https://tomorrowhealthcare.org/full-consultation-with-patrick
5. https://www.skype.com/en/download-skype/skype-for-computer/
6. https://www.whatsapp.com/download/

REIKI SHOP

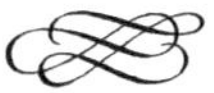

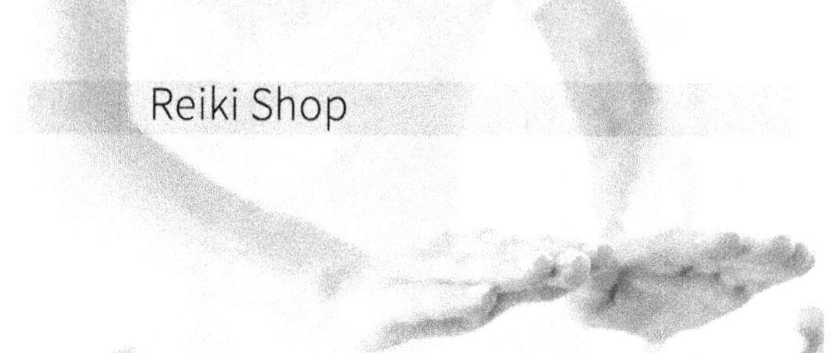

REIKI MP3 MUSIC SHOP

Full Reiki Shop[1]

REIKI MEDITATION TO MEET YOUR REIKI GUIDE — MP3 FORMAT TO DOWNLOAD.

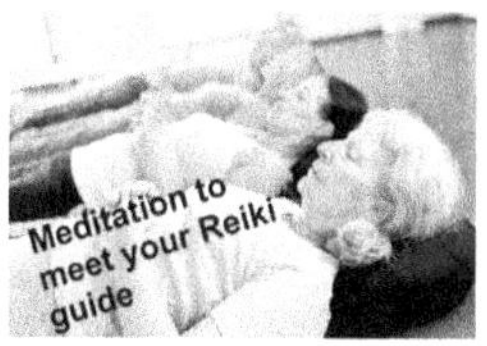

Purchase the above here[2]

---

1. https://tomorrowhealthcare.org/reiki-healing-shop
2. Reiki Meditation to Meet your Guide: https://tomorrowhealthcare.org/meet-your-reiki-guide

REIKI MUSIC WITH TIBETAN BELL EVERY 3 MINUTES — MP3 FORMAT TO DOWNLOAD.

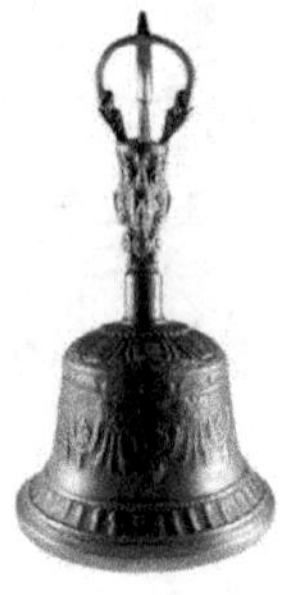

MP3 available in my shop

Gentle background Reiki music with a warning to move your hands every 3 minutes — MP3 format to download.

Purchase Tibetan Bell every 3 minutes here[3]

GENTLE MUSIC WITH A WHISPERED WARNING TO MOVE YOUR HANDS EVERY 3 MINUTES

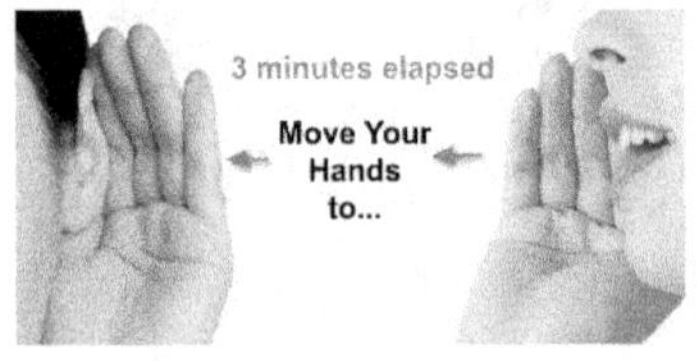

MP3 available in my shop

Purchase Music with gentle warning here[4]

---

3. http://tomorrowhealthcare.org/purchase-tibetan-bell-3-minutes
4. https://tomorrowhealthcare.org/reiki-music-with-hand-position

ALL THREE REIKI INITIATIONS ON VIDEO

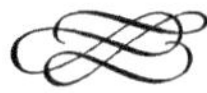

Reiki Shop

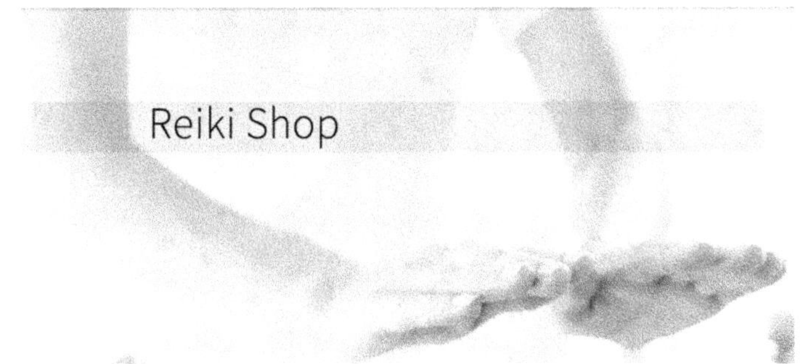

ALL *REIKI INITIATIONS CAPTURED ON VIDEO* — AVAILABLE TO DOWNLOAD.

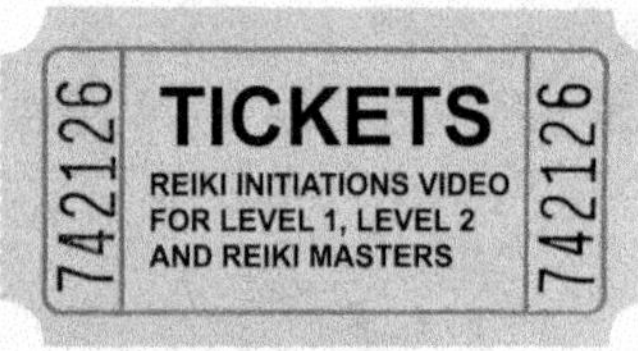

This movie is available in my shop

ALL THREE REIKI MANUALS

<u>Reiki Shop</u>[1]

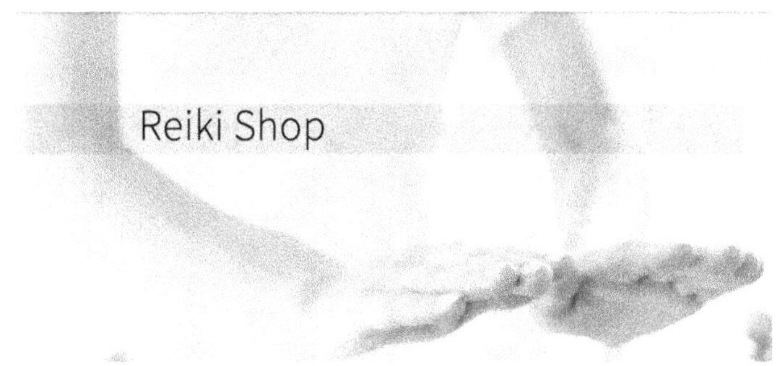

---

1. Reiki Shop: https://tomorrowhealthcare.org/reiki-healing-shop

REIKI MANUALS FOR REIKI 1, REIKI 2 AND REIKI MASTER.

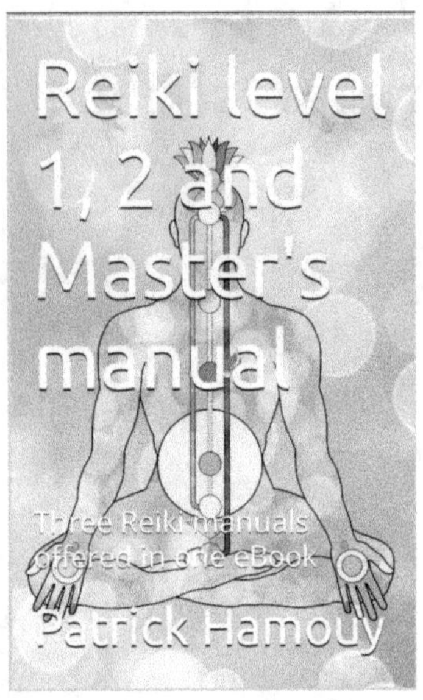

All three Reiki manuals available in my shop

Symbols

D

E

F

learn the different levels
of reiki in two
weekends[1], 45
light struck him on the
third eye[1], 17
listen to your hand.[1],
70

M

master[2], 5, 90
master passes on reiki
to a student[1], 47
mental/emotional
symbol[1], 74
mikaomi[1], 21
mikaomi usui[2], 3, 21
minutes[1], 86
mount kurama waterfall
is where usui
meditated[1], 22
mountain of koriyama
[1], 16
murmur a prayer[1], 59
my clairvoyant friend[2],
4, 52

N

nergy amplification[1],
50

O

ogawa[1], 21
operation is not
necessary[1], 27
origin of reiki[1], 9

P

patrick hamouy[1], 77
patrick specialises in[1],
77
phyllis furumoto is
takata's
granddaughter[1],
30
power symbol[1], 74
presidents were[1], 23
principal of doshisha
university[1], 14

R

radiance technique[1],
32
rei means[1], 10
reiki 2[1], 74
reiki 3 gives you access
to the master
symbol[1], 75
reiki alliance[1], 35
reiki can never cause
harm[1], 46